"NO MATTER HOW LITTLE MONEY AND HOW FEW POSSESSIONS YOU OWN, HAVING A DOG MAKES YOU RICH"

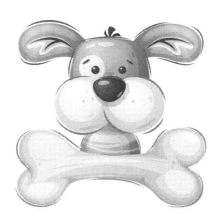

TABLE OF CONTENTS

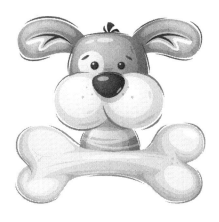

Thank you for purchasing this book!
If you like it, we would appreciate your review on Amazon.
That way, we could improve our work, and other customers
would buy with confidence.

If you would like
a birth certificate or an adoption certificate for your dog,
as PDF printable freebie, just contact us at:
GoodX2Come@outlook.de

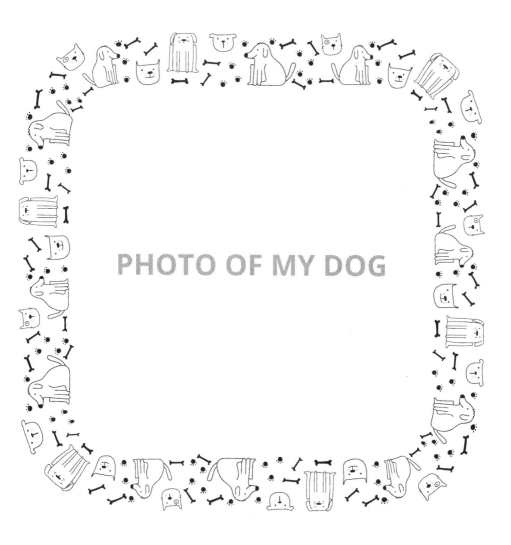

PHOTO OF MY DOG

DOG *Information*

NAME	
BIRTHDAY	
BREED	
GENDER	
COAT COLOR	
EYE COLOR	
ADOPTION DATE / PLACE	
SPECIAL MARKINGS	
WEIGHT & HIGHT	
PARENTS INFORMATION	
ALLERGIES	
MEDIACL CONDITION	
ILLNES	
SPAYED / NEUTERED	
MICROCHIP COMPANY	
MICROCHIP ID	
INSURANCE COMPANY	
POLICY TYPE / NUMBER	
INSURANCE CONTACT	

OWNER *Information*

NAME	
ADDRESS	
PHONE	
MOBILE	
EMAIL	

VET *Information*

NAME	
ADDRESS	
PHONE	
MOBILE	
EMAIL	

NAME	
ADDRESS	
PHONE	
MOBILE	
EMAIL	

NAME	
ADDRESS	
PHONE	
MOBILE	
EMAIL	

PET CLINIC *Information*

HOSPITAL NAME	
ADDRESS	
PHONE	
MOBILE	
EMAIL	

DOG SERVICE *Information*

GROOMING CENTER	
ADDRESS	
PHONE	
MOBILE	
EMAIL	

DOG SITTER NAME	
MOBILE	
EMAIL	

DOG SITTER NAME	
MOBILE	
EMAIL	

ANIMAL SHELTER	
ADDRESS	
PHONE	
MOBILE	
EMAIL	

TRAINING CENTER	
MOBILE	
EMAIL	

TRAINER NAME	
MOBILE	
EMAIL	

DOG DEVELOPMENT *Information*

AGE	WEIGHT & HIGHT	DATE	OBSERVATION
8 WEEKS		___/___/___	
12 WEEKS		___/___/___	
16 WEEKS		___/___/___	
20 WEEKS		___/___/___	
6 MONTHS		___/___/___	
1 YEAR		___/___/___	
2 YEARS		___/___/___	
3 YEARS		___/___/___	
4 YEARS		___/___/___	
5 YEARS		___/___/___	
6 YEARS		___/___/___	
7 YEARS		___/___/___	
8 YEARS		___/___/___	
9 YEARS		___/___/___	
10 YEARS		___/___/___	
11 YEARS		___/___/___	
12 YEARS		___/___/___	
13 YEARS		___/___/___	
14 YEARS		___/___/___	
15 YEARS		___/___/___	
16 YEARS		___/___/___	
17 YEARS		___/___/___	
18 YEARS		___/___/___	
19 YEARS		___/___/___	
20 YEARS		___/___/___	

DOG TRAINING *Information*

DATE	TRAINING
___/___/___	
___/___/___	
___/___/___	
___/___/___	
___/___/___	
___/___/___	
___/___/___	
___/___/___	
___/___/___	
___/___/___	
___/___/___	
___/___/___	
___/___/___	
___/___/___	
___/___/___	
___/___/___	
___/___/___	
___/___/___	
___/___/___	
___/___/___	
___/___/___	
___/___/___	
___/___/___	

VACCINATIONS *Information*

BORDETELLA

DATE	DATE	DATE	DATE
___/___/___	___/___/___	___/___/___	___/___/___
___/___/___	___/___/___	___/___/___	___/___/___
___/___/___	___/___/___	___/___/___	___/___/___

Bordetella bronchiseptica is a bacterium that is associated with respiratory disease in dogs. It is one of the components of the canine infectious respiratory complex, sometimes referred to as kennel cough, upper respiratory infection, or infectious tracheobronchitis.

DISTEMPER

DATE	DATE	DATE	DATE
___/___/___	___/___/___	___/___/___	___/___/___
___/___/___	___/___/___	___/___/___	___/___/___
___/___/___	___/___/___	___/___/___	___/___/___

Canine distemper is a contagious and serious disease caused by a virus that attacks the respiratory, gastrointestinal and nervous systems of puppies and dogs. Puppies and dogs most often become infected through airborne exposure (through sneezing or coughing) to the virus from an infected dog or wild animal.

CORONAVIRUS

DATE	DATE	DATE	DATE
___/___/___	___/___/___	___/___/___	___/___/___
___/___/___	___/___/___	___/___/___	___/___/___
___/___/___	___/___/___	___/___/___	___/___/___

Canine coronavirus disease, known as CCoV, is a highly infectious intestinal infection in dogs, especially puppies. Canine coronavirus is usually short-lived but may cause considerable abdominal discomfort for a few days in infected dogs.

HEPATITIS / ADENOVIRUS

DATE	DATE	DATE	DATE
___/___/___	___/___/___	___/___/___	___/___/___
___/___/___	___/___/___	___/___/___	___/___/___
___/___/___	___/___/___	___/___/___	___/___/___

Infectious canine hepatitis is an acute contagious disease caused by the canine adenovirus 1. This virus targets the spleen, kidneys, lungs, liver, lining of blood vessels and sometimes other organs. Symptoms can vary widely - from slight fever, thirst or apathy to death.

LEPTOSPIROSIS

DATE	DATE	DATE	DATE
___/___/___	___/___/___	___/___/___	___/___/___
___/___/___	___/___/___	___/___/___	___/___/___
___/___/___	___/___/___	___/___/___	___/___/___

Leptospirosis is a bacterial disease of dogs and other mammals that primarily affects the liver or kidneys. The bacteria (Leptospira) that cause leptospirosis, commonly called leptospires, thrive in water. Infected or recovered carrier dogs may act as a source of the infection.

PARVOVIRUS

DATE	DATE	DATE	DATE
___/___/___	___/___/___	___/___/___	___/___/___
___/___/___	___/___/___	___/___/___	___/___/___
___/___/___	___/___/___	___/___/___	___/___/___

The clinical signs and symptoms of CPV disease can vary, but generally they include severe vomiting and diarrhea. The virus is easily transmitted via the hair or feet of infected dogs, or on shoes, clothes, and other objects contaminated by infected feces.

PARAINFLUENZA

DATE	DATE	DATE	DATE
___/___/___	___/___/___	___/___/___	___/___/___
___/___/___	___/___/___	___/___/___	___/___/___
___/___/___	___/___/___	___/___/___	___/___/___

Canine parainfluenza virus (CPIV) is a highly contagious respiratory virus and is one of the most common pathogens of infectious tracheobronchitis, also known as canine cough.3Although the respiratory signs may resemble those of canine influenza, they are unrelated viruses and require different vaccines for protection.

RABIES

DATE	DATE	DATE	DATE
___/___/___	___/___/___	___/___/___	___/___/___
___/___/___	___/___/___	___/___/___	___/___/___
___/___/___	___/___/___	___/___/___	___/___/___

Rabies is one of the deadliest diseases affecting animals, and dogs are no exception. As there is no cure for rabies, keeping up with regular vaccinations is essential. Once a dog is infected, the virus progresses rapidly. It usually takes less than 10 days to develop, but it can take up to one year.

CANINE INFLUENZA

DATE	DATE	DATE	DATE
___/___/___	___/___/___	___/___/___	___/___/___
___/___/___	___/___/___	___/___/___	___/___/___
___/___/___	___/___/___	___/___/___	___/___/___

Canine influenza virus (CIV) is primarily the result of two influenza strains: H3N8 from an equine origin and H3N2 from an avian origin. The symptoms of canine influenza are similar to the human flu: cough, runny nose, and fever.

HEARTWORM PREVENTION DATES

DATE	DATE	DATE	DATE
...../...../.....	...../...../.....	...../...../.....	...../...../.....
...../...../.....	...../...../.....	...../...../.....	...../...../.....
...../...../.....	...../...../.....	...../...../.....	...../...../.....
...../...../.....	...../...../.....	...../...../.....	...../...../.....
...../...../.....	...../...../.....	...../...../.....	...../...../.....
...../...../.....	...../...../.....	...../...../.....	...../...../.....
...../...../.....	...../...../.....	...../...../.....	...../...../.....
...../...../.....	...../...../.....	...../...../.....	...../...../.....
...../...../.....	...../...../.....	...../...../.....	...../...../.....

FLEA & TICK PREVENTION DATES

DATE	DATE	DATE	DATE
...../...../.....	...../...../.....	...../...../.....	...../...../.....
...../...../.....	...../...../.....	...../...../.....	...../...../.....
...../...../.....	...../...../.....	...../...../.....	...../...../.....
...../...../.....	...../...../.....	...../...../.....	...../...../.....
...../...../.....	...../...../.....	...../...../.....	...../...../.....
...../...../.....	...../...../.....	...../...../.....	...../...../.....
...../...../.....	...../...../.....	...../...../.....	...../...../.....
...../...../.....	...../...../.....	...../...../.....	...../...../.....
...../...../.....	...../...../.....	...../...../.....	...../...../.....
...../...../.....	...../...../.....	...../...../.....	...../...../.....

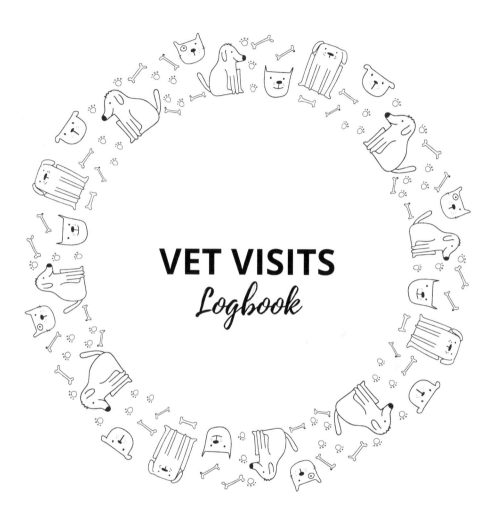

VET VISITS
Logbook

VET VISIT LOG

DATE /TIME	
KIND OF VISIT	ROUTINE ☐ EMERGENCY ☐
SHOTS	
MEDICATION	
OTHER TREATMENT	
COMMENTS	
COST	

DATE /TIME	
KIND OF VISIT	ROUTINE ☐ EMERGENCY ☐
SHOTS	
MEDICATION	
OTHER TREATMENT	
COMMENTS	
COST	

VET VISIT LOG

DATE /TIME	
KIND OF VISIT	ROUTINE ☐ EMERGENCY ☐
SHOTS	
MEDICATION	
OTHER TREATMENT	
COMMENTS	
COST	

DATE /TIME	
KIND OF VISIT	ROUTINE ☐ EMERGENCY ☐
SHOTS	
MEDICATION	
OTHER TREATMENT	
COMMENTS	
COST	

VET VISIT LOG

DATE /TIME	
KIND OF VISIT	ROUTINE ☐ EMERGENCY ☐
SHOTS	
MEDICATION	
OTHER TREATMENT	
COMMENTS	
COST	

DATE /TIME	
KIND OF VISIT	ROUTINE ☐ EMERGENCY ☐
SHOTS	
MEDICATION	
OTHER TREATMENT	
COMMENTS	
COST	

VET VISIT LOG

DATE /TIME	
KIND OF VISIT	ROUTINE ☐ EMERGENCY ☐
SHOTS	
MEDICATION	
OTHER TREATMENT	
COMMENTS	
COST	

DATE /TIME	
KIND OF VISIT	ROUTINE ☐ EMERGENCY ☐
SHOTS	
MEDICATION	
OTHER TREATMENT	
COMMENTS	
COST	

VET VISIT LOG

DATE /TIME	
KIND OF VISIT	ROUTINE ☐　　EMERGENCY ☐
SHOTS	
MEDICATION	
OTHER TREATMENT	
COMMENTS	
COST	

DATE /TIME	
KIND OF VISIT	ROUTINE ☐　　EMERGENCY ☐
SHOTS	
MEDICATION	
OTHER TREATMENT	
COMMENTS	
COST	

VET VISIT LOG

DATE /TIME	
KIND OF VISIT	ROUTINE ☐ EMERGENCY ☐
SHOTS	
MEDICATION	
OTHER TREATMENT	
COMMENTS	
COST	

DATE /TIME	
KIND OF VISIT	ROUTINE ☐ EMERGENCY ☐
SHOTS	
MEDICATION	
OTHER TREATMENT	
COMMENTS	
COST	

VET VISIT LOG

DATE /TIME	
KIND OF VISIT	ROUTINE ☐ EMERGENCY ☐
SHOTS	
MEDICATION	
OTHER TREATMENT	
COMMENTS	
COST	

DATE /TIME	
KIND OF VISIT	ROUTINE ☐ EMERGENCY ☐
SHOTS	
MEDICATION	
OTHER TREATMENT	
COMMENTS	
COST	

VET VISIT LOG

DATE /TIME	
KIND OF VISIT	ROUTINE ☐ EMERGENCY ☐
SHOTS	
MEDICATION	
OTHER TREATMENT	
COMMENTS	
COST	

DATE /TIME	
KIND OF VISIT	ROUTINE ☐ EMERGENCY ☐
SHOTS	
MEDICATION	
OTHER TREATMENT	
COMMENTS	
COST	

VET VISIT LOG

DATE /TIME	
KIND OF VISIT	ROUTINE ☐ EMERGENCY ☐
SHOTS	
MEDICATION	
OTHER TREATMENT	
COMMENTS	
COST	

DATE /TIME	
KIND OF VISIT	ROUTINE ☐ EMERGENCY ☐
SHOTS	
MEDICATION	
OTHER TREATMENT	
COMMENTS	
COST	

VET VISIT LOG

DATE /TIME	
KIND OF VISIT	ROUTINE ☐ EMERGENCY ☐
SHOTS	
MEDICATION	
OTHER TREATMENT	
COMMENTS	
COST	

DATE /TIME	
KIND OF VISIT	ROUTINE ☐ EMERGENCY ☐
SHOTS	
MEDICATION	
OTHER TREATMENT	
COMMENTS	
COST	

VET VISIT LOG

DATE /TIME	
KIND OF VISIT	ROUTINE ☐ EMERGENCY ☐
SHOTS	
MEDICATION	
OTHER TREATMENT	
COMMENTS	
COST	

DATE /TIME	
KIND OF VISIT	ROUTINE ☐ EMERGENCY ☐
SHOTS	
MEDICATION	
OTHER TREATMENT	
COMMENTS	
COST	

VET VISIT LOG

DATE /TIME	
KIND OF VISIT	ROUTINE ☐ EMERGENCY ☐
SHOTS	
MEDICATION	
OTHER TREATMENT	
COMMENTS	
COST	

DATE /TIME	
KIND OF VISIT	ROUTINE ☐ EMERGENCY ☐
SHOTS	
MEDICATION	
OTHER TREATMENT	
COMMENTS	
COST	

VET VISIT LOG

DATE /TIME	
KIND OF VISIT	ROUTINE ☐ EMERGENCY ☐
SHOTS	
MEDICATION	
OTHER TREATMENT	
COMMENTS	
COST	

DATE /TIME	
KIND OF VISIT	ROUTINE ☐ EMERGENCY ☐
SHOTS	
MEDICATION	
OTHER TREATMENT	
COMMENTS	
COST	

28

VET VISIT LOG

DATE /TIME	
KIND OF VISIT	ROUTINE ☐ EMERGENCY ☐
SHOTS	
MEDICATION	
OTHER TREATMENT	
COMMENTS	
COST	

DATE /TIME	
KIND OF VISIT	ROUTINE ☐ EMERGENCY ☐
SHOTS	
MEDICATION	
OTHER TREATMENT	
COMMENTS	
COST	

VET VISIT LOG

DATE /TIME	
KIND OF VISIT	ROUTINE ☐ EMERGENCY ☐
SHOTS	
MEDICATION	
OTHER TREATMENT	
COMMENTS	
COST	

DATE /TIME	
KIND OF VISIT	ROUTINE ☐ EMERGENCY ☐
SHOTS	
MEDICATION	
OTHER TREATMENT	
COMMENTS	
COST	

VET VISIT LOG

DATE /TIME	
KIND OF VISIT	ROUTINE ☐ EMERGENCY ☐
SHOTS	
MEDICATION	
OTHER TREATMENT	
COMMENTS	
COST	

DATE /TIME	
KIND OF VISIT	ROUTINE ☐ EMERGENCY ☐
SHOTS	
MEDICATION	
OTHER TREATMENT	
COMMENTS	
COST	

VET VISIT LOG

DATE /TIME	
KIND OF VISIT	ROUTINE ☐ EMERGENCY ☐
SHOTS	
MEDICATION	
OTHER TREATMENT	
COMMENTS	
COST	

DATE /TIME	
KIND OF VISIT	ROUTINE ☐ EMERGENCY ☐
SHOTS	
MEDICATION	
OTHER TREATMENT	
COMMENTS	
COST	

VET VISIT LOG

DATE /TIME	
KIND OF VISIT	ROUTINE ☐ EMERGENCY ☐
SHOTS	
MEDICATION	
OTHER TREATMENT	
COMMENTS	
COST	

DATE /TIME	
KIND OF VISIT	ROUTINE ☐ EMERGENCY ☐
SHOTS	
MEDICATION	
OTHER TREATMENT	
COMMENTS	
COST	

VET VISIT LOG

DATE /TIME	
KIND OF VISIT	ROUTINE ☐ EMERGENCY ☐
SHOTS	
MEDICATION	
OTHER TREATMENT	
COMMENTS	
COST	

DATE /TIME	
KIND OF VISIT	ROUTINE ☐ EMERGENCY ☐
SHOTS	
MEDICATION	
OTHER TREATMENT	
COMMENTS	
COST	

34

VET VISIT LOG

DATE / TIME	
KIND OF VISIT	ROUTINE ☐ EMERGENCY ☐
SHOTS	
MEDICATION	
OTHER TREATMENT	
COMMENTS	
COST	

DATE / TIME	
KIND OF VISIT	ROUTINE ☐ EMERGENCY ☐
SHOTS	
MEDICATION	
OTHER TREATMENT	
COMMENTS	
COST	

VET VISIT LOG

DATE /TIME	
KIND OF VISIT	ROUTINE ☐ EMERGENCY ☐
SHOTS	
MEDICATION	
OTHER TREATMENT	
COMMENTS	
COST	

DATE /TIME	
KIND OF VISIT	ROUTINE ☐ EMERGENCY ☐
SHOTS	
MEDICATION	
OTHER TREATMENT	
COMMENTS	
COST	

VET VISIT LOG

DATE /TIME	
KIND OF VISIT	ROUTINE ☐ EMERGENCY ☐
SHOTS	
MEDICATION	
OTHER TREATMENT	
COMMENTS	
COST	

DATE /TIME	
KIND OF VISIT	ROUTINE ☐ EMERGENCY ☐
SHOTS	
MEDICATION	
OTHER TREATMENT	
COMMENTS	
COST	

VET VISIT LOG

DATE /TIME	
KIND OF VISIT	ROUTINE ☐ EMERGENCY ☐
SHOTS	
MEDICATION	
OTHER TREATMENT	
COMMENTS	
COST	

DATE /TIME	
KIND OF VISIT	ROUTINE ☐ EMERGENCY ☐
SHOTS	
MEDICATION	
OTHER TREATMENT	
COMMENTS	
COST	

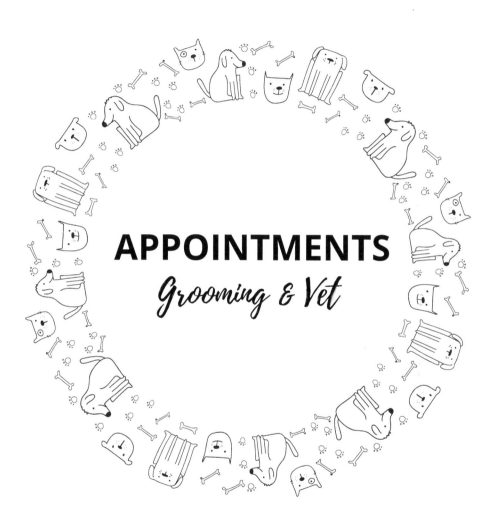

APPOINTMENTS
Grooming & Vet

APPOINTMENTS *Grooming*

DATE	NOTES
___/___/___	
___/___/___	
___/___/___	
___/___/___	
___/___/___	
___/___/___	
___/___/___	
___/___/___	
___/___/___	
___/___/___	
___/___/___	
___/___/___	
___/___/___	
___/___/___	
___/___/___	
___/___/___	
___/___/___	
___/___/___	
___/___/___	
___/___/___	
___/___/___	
___/___/___	
___/___/___	

APPOINTMENTS *Grooming*

DATE	NOTES
___/___/___	
___/___/___	
___/___/___	
___/___/___	
___/___/___	
___/___/___	
___/___/___	
___/___/___	
___/___/___	
___/___/___	
___/___/___	
___/___/___	
___/___/___	
___/___/___	
___/___/___	
___/___/___	
___/___/___	
___/___/___	
___/___/___	
___/___/___	
___/___/___	
___/___/___	
___/___/___	
___/___/___	
___/___/___	

APPOINTMENTS *Veterinarian*

DATE	NOTES
___/___/___	
___/___/___	
___/___/___	
___/___/___	
___/___/___	
___/___/___	
___/___/___	
___/___/___	
___/___/___	
___/___/___	
___/___/___	
___/___/___	
___/___/___	
___/___/___	
___/___/___	
___/___/___	
___/___/___	
___/___/___	
___/___/___	
___/___/___	
___/___/___	
___/___/___	
___/___/___	

APPOINTMENTS *Veterinarian*

DATE	NOTES
___/___/___	
___/___/___	
___/___/___	
___/___/___	
___/___/___	
___/___/___	
___/___/___	
___/___/___	
___/___/___	
___/___/___	
___/___/___	
___/___/___	
___/___/___	
___/___/___	
___/___/___	
___/___/___	
___/___/___	
___/___/___	
___/___/___	
___/___/___	
___/___/___	
___/___/___	
___/___/___	
___/___/___	
___/___/___	

NOTES

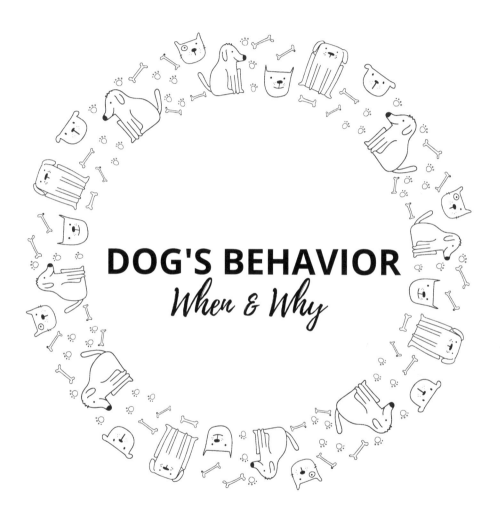

DOG'S BEHAVIOR
When & Why

BEHAVIOR *Information*

TYPE	WHEN	WHY
BARKING		
CHEWING		
DIGGING		
BEGGING		
CHASING		
JUMPING UP		
BITING		
LICKING		
AGGRESSION		
ROLLICK ABOUT		
ANXIETY		
LONG SLEEP		
YAWNING		

MY DOG LIKES

TOYS

TREATS

HUMANS / CREATURES

OUTINGS

MY DOG DOESN'T LIKE

WEATHER

PLACES

HUMANS / CREATURES

GESTURES & SOUNDS

MY DOG'S FEEDING PREFERENCES

DRIED FOOD

WET FOOD

SNACKS

DRINKS

MY DOG'S WALKING & CLOTHING PREFERENCES

WALKING

CLOTHES & SHOES

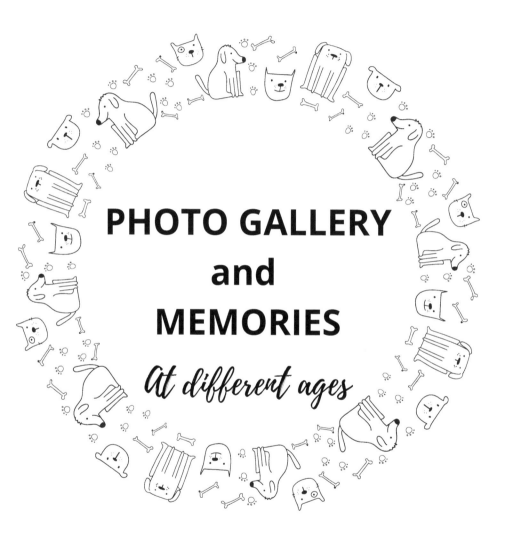

PHOTO GALLERY
and
MEMORIES
At different ages

MEMORIES & NOTES

At 8 weeks

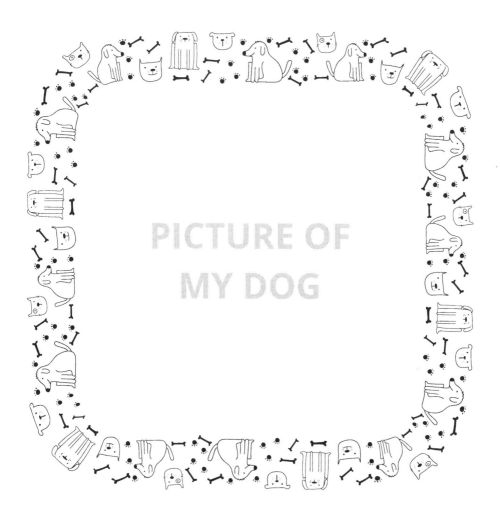

PICTURE OF
MY DOG

DATE:

PLACE:

EVENT:

MEMORIES & NOTES

At 12 weeks

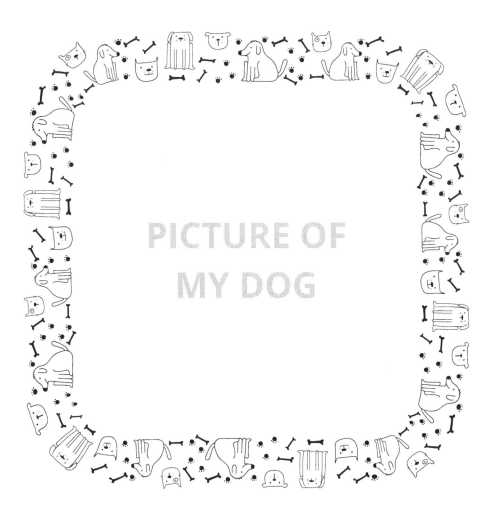

PICTURE OF
MY DOG

DATE:

PLACE:

EVENT:

MEMORIES & NOTES

At 16 weeks

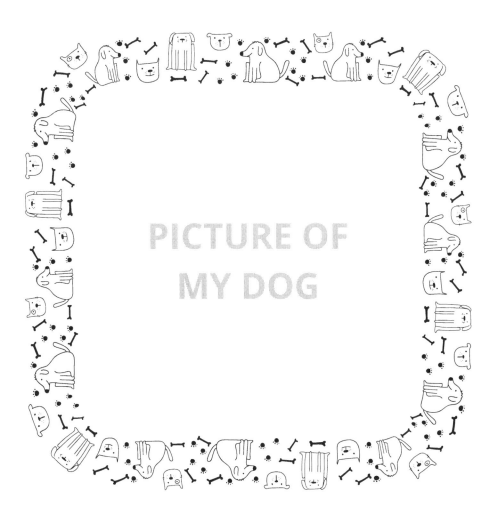

PICTURE OF
MY DOG

DATE:

PLACE:

EVENT:

MEMORIES & NOTES

At 20 weeks

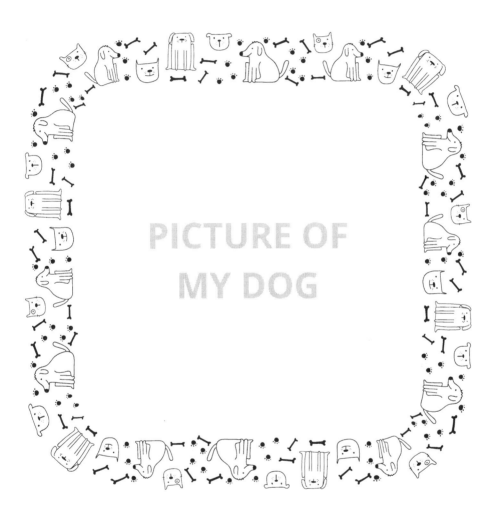

PICTURE OF
MY DOG

DATE:

PLACE:

EVENT:

MEMORIES & NOTES

At 6 months

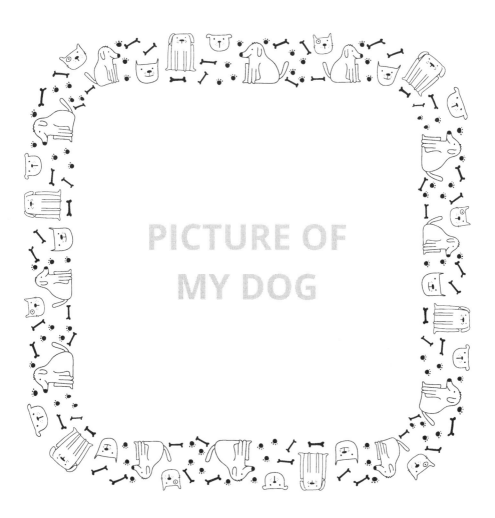

PICTURE OF
MY DOG

DATE:

PLACE:

EVENT:

MEMORIES & NOTES

At 1 year

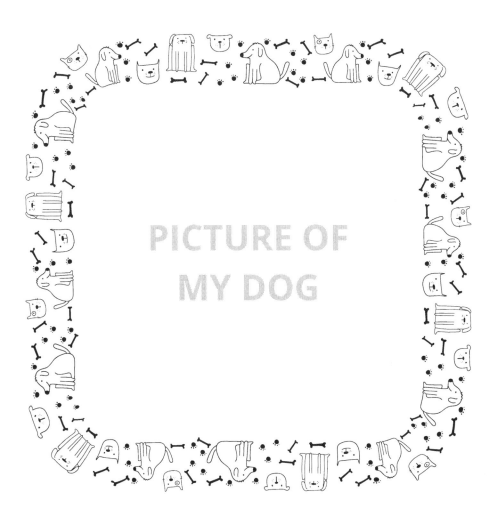

PICTURE OF
MY DOG

DATE:

PLACE:

EVENT:

MEMORIES & NOTES

At 2 years

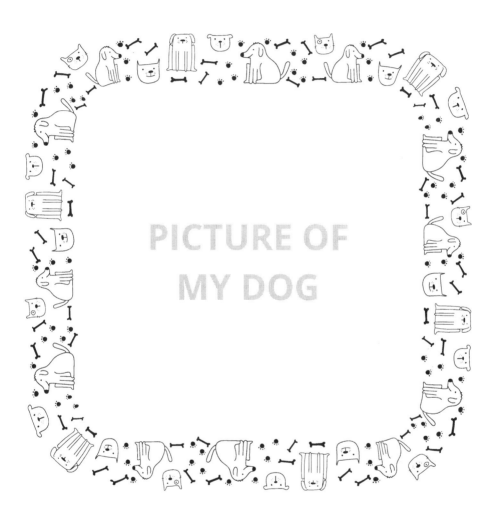

PICTURE OF
MY DOG

DATE:
PLACE:
EVENT:

MEMORIES & NOTES

At 3 years

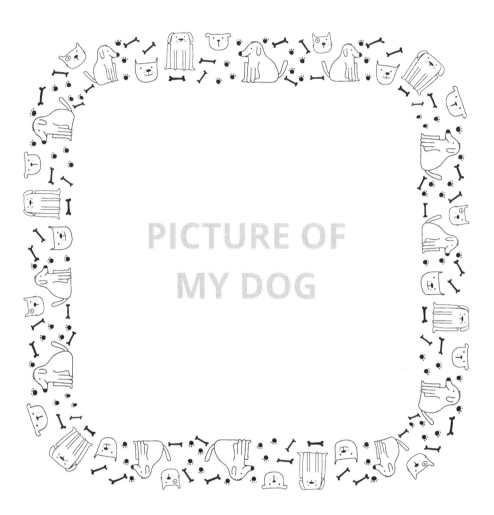

PICTURE OF
MY DOG

DATE:
PLACE:
EVENT:

MEMORIES & NOTES

At 4 years

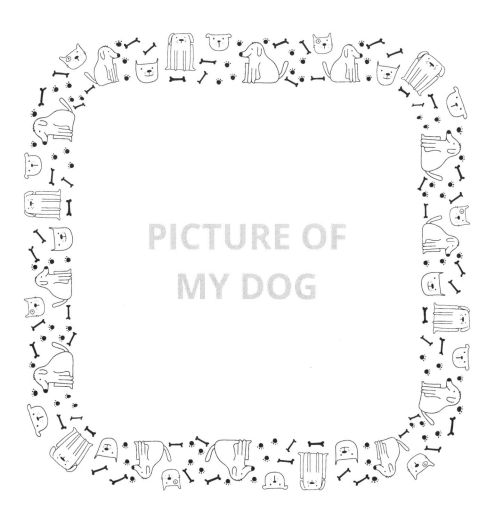

PICTURE OF
MY DOG

DATE:
PLACE:
EVENT:

MEMORIES & NOTES

At 5 years

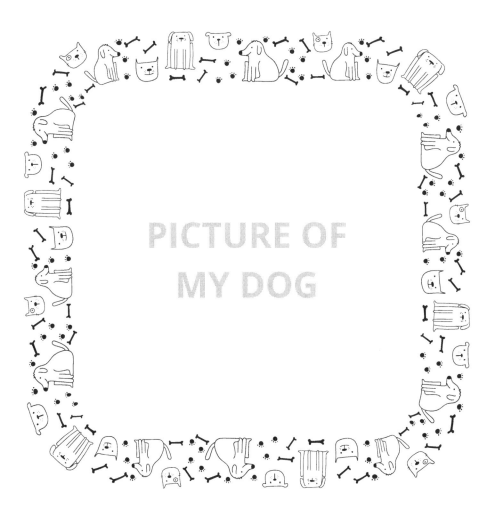

PICTURE OF
MY DOG

DATE:

PLACE:

EVENT:

MEMORIES & NOTES

At 6 years

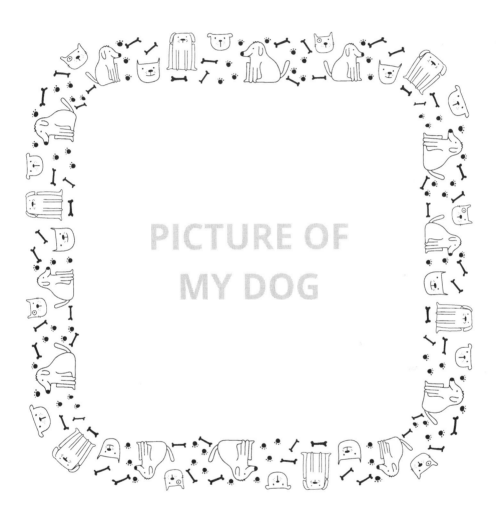

PICTURE OF
MY DOG

DATE:
PLACE:
EVENT:

MEMORIES & NOTES

At 7 years

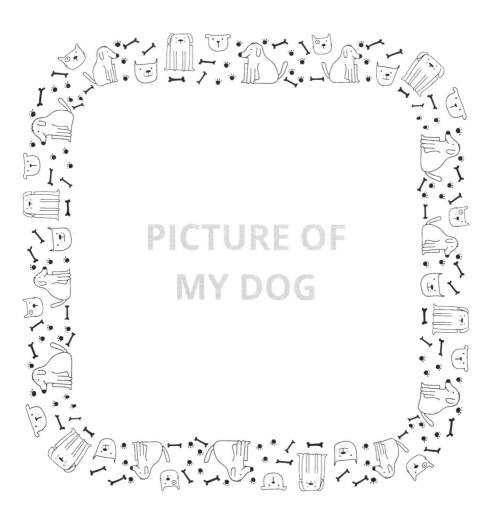

PICTURE OF
MY DOG

DATE:

PLACE:

EVENT:

MEMORIES & NOTES

At 8 years

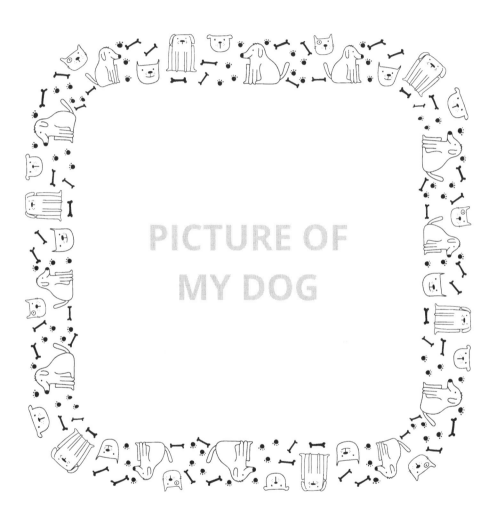

PICTURE OF
MY DOG

DATE:

PLACE:

EVENT:

MEMORIES & NOTES

At 9 years

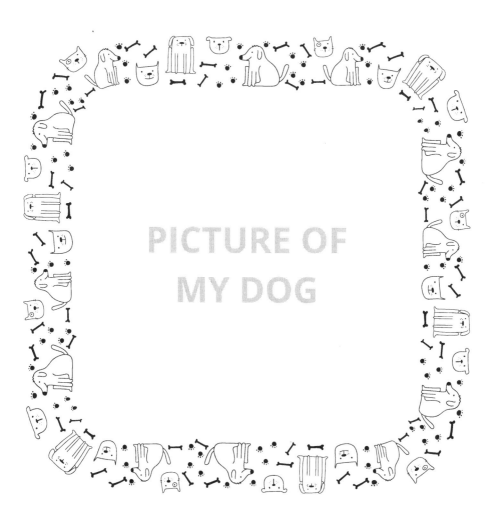

PICTURE OF
MY DOG

DATE:

PLACE:

EVENT:

MEMORIES & NOTES

At 10 years

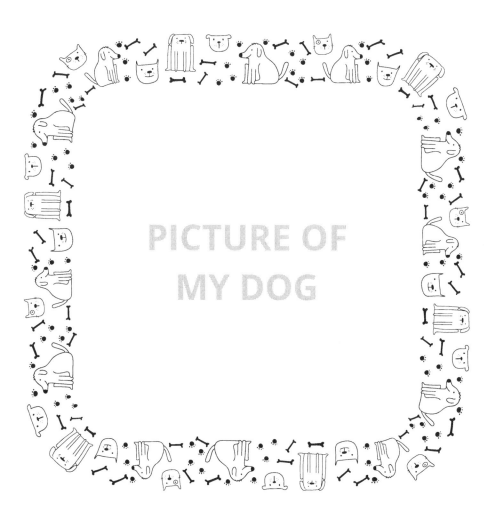

PICTURE OF
MY DOG

DATE:

PLACE:

EVENT:

MEMORIES & NOTES

At 11 years

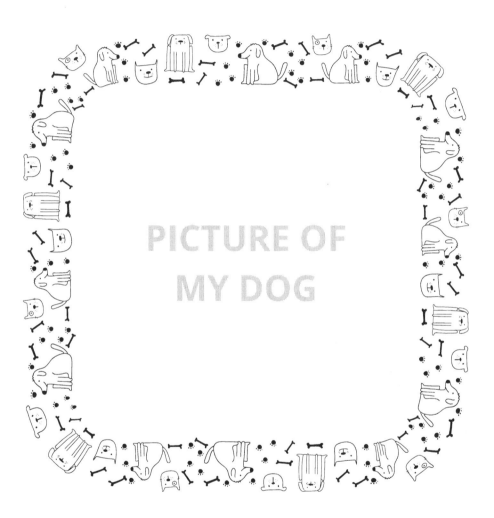

PICTURE OF
MY DOG

DATE:

PLACE:

EVENT:

MEMORIES & NOTES

At 12 years

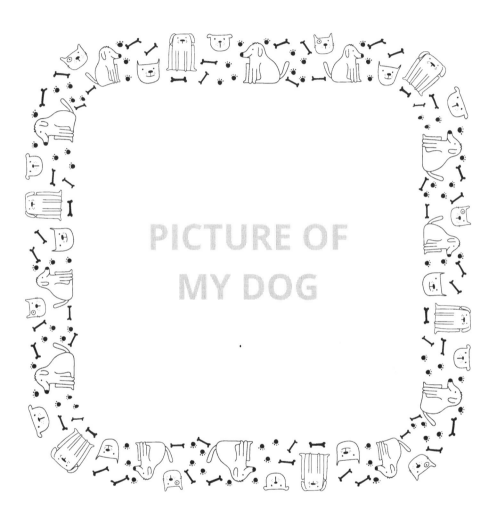

PICTURE OF
MY DOG

DATE:

PLACE:

EVENT:

MEMORIES & NOTES

At 13 years

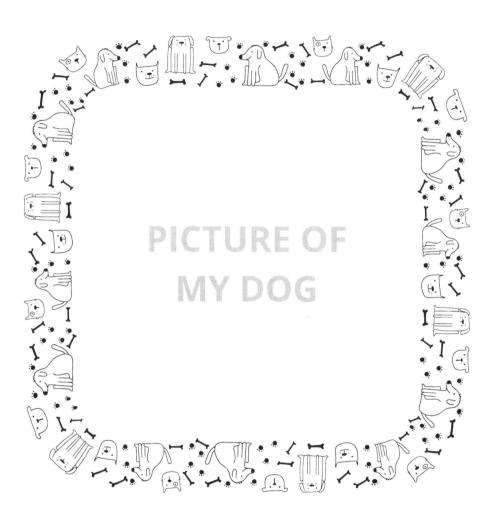

PICTURE OF
MY DOG

DATE:
PLACE:
EVENT:

MEMORIES & NOTES

At 14 years

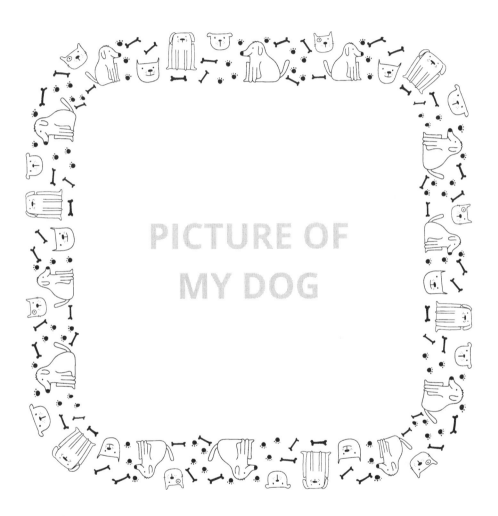

PICTURE OF
MY DOG

DATE:
PLACE:
EVENT:

MEMORIES & NOTES

At 15 years

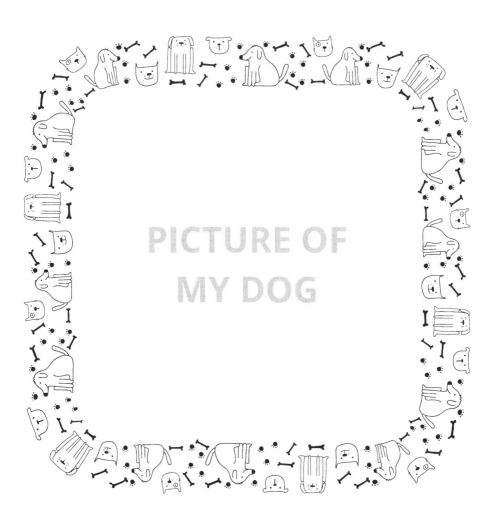

PICTURE OF
MY DOG

DATE:

PLACE:

EVENT:

MEMORIES & NOTES

At 16 years

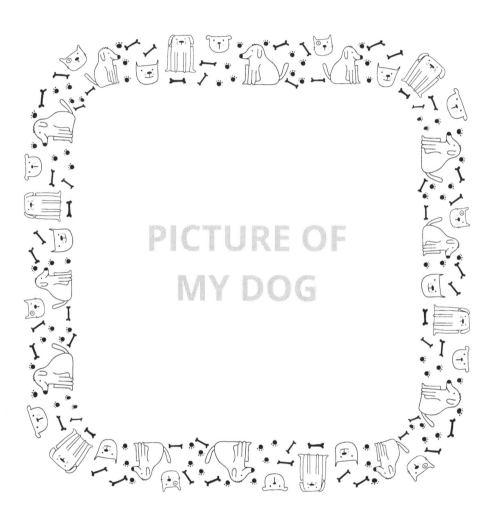

PICTURE OF
MY DOG

DATE:

PLACE:

EVENT:

MEMORIES & NOTES

At 17 years

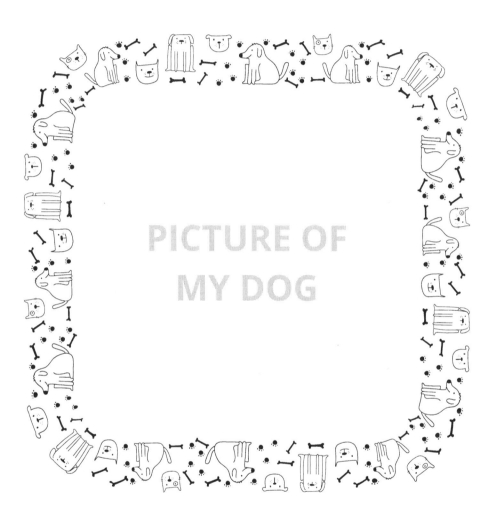

PICTURE OF
MY DOG

DATE:

PLACE:

EVENT:

MEMORIES & NOTES

At 18 years

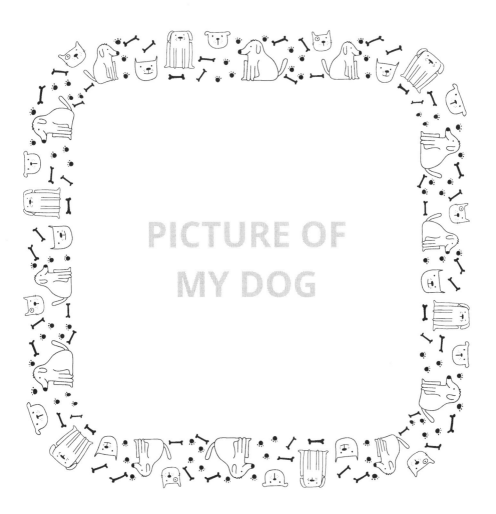

PICTURE OF
MY DOG

DATE:

PLACE:

EVENT:

MEMORIES & NOTES

At 19 years

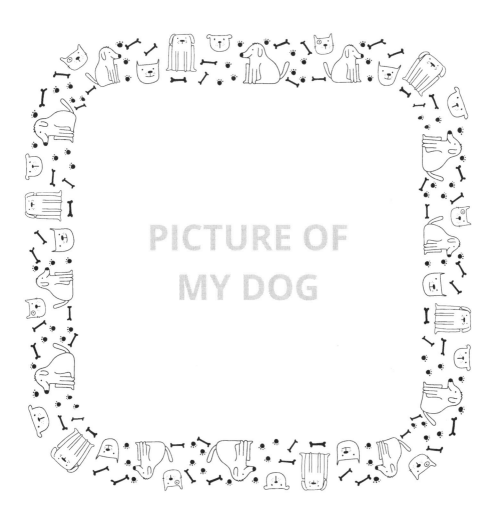

PICTURE OF
MY DOG

DATE:

PLACE:

EVENT:

MEMORIES & NOTES

At 20 years

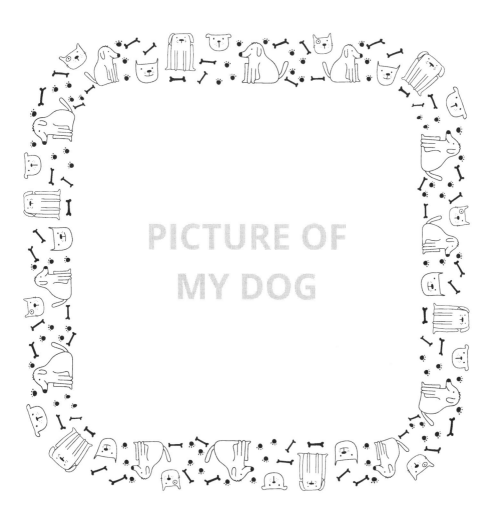

PICTURE OF
MY DOG

DATE:

PLACE:

EVENT:

NOTES

NOTES

NOTES

Made in the USA
Monee, IL
02 December 2022

19314383R00059